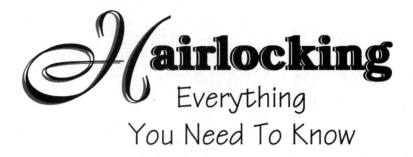

Hairlocking
Everything You Need To Know

AFRICAN, DREAD & NUBIAN LOCKS

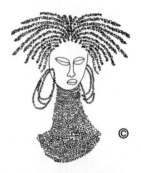

NEW BEIN' ENTERPRISES

Published by
A&B Publishers Group
Brooklyn, New York

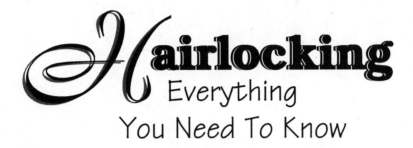

Hairlocking
Everything You Need To Know

AFRICAN, DREAD & NUBIAN LOCKS

Nekhena Evans

Published by
A&B Publishers Group
Brooklyn, New York

COVER DESIGN: *A & B PUBLISHER GROUP*
COVER PHOTO: *PRESTON PHILLIPS*

Library of Congress Cataloging-in-Publication Data

Evans, Nekhena.
        Everything you need to know about hairlocking, African, dread & nubian locks/ Nekhena Evans /3 rd ed.
        p.   cm.
        Includes bibliographical references and index.
        ISBN 1-886433-15-1
        1. Dreadlocks 2. Hairdressing of Blacks 3. Braids (Hairdressing). 4.
Hairstyles.   I. Title.
GT2290.E93   1998   98-15601
646. 7'24' --dc21   CIP

Published
by

A&B PUBLISHERS GROUP
1000 Atlantic Avenue
Brooklyn, New York,
    •   11238
(718) 783-7808
01 02   7 6 5

Manufactured and Printed in the United States

Dedication

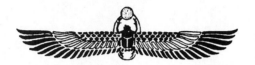

THIS WORK IS DEDICATED TO the Creator with whom I am one. I give him thanks and praise for allowing me to be a servant through my work. I further dedicate this book to my ancestors and to those yet unborn; to my parents, Ralph and Frezell Evans and to my children Nadira and Nile whom I love dearly. I hope this work serves as a source of pride and inspiration. I must also commend my devotion to my mentor Sayini Morningstar, who taught me the tradition of hairlocking, and to the memory of Karima, a friend and beautiful sister who touched many lives as a locktician.

Ashe'

Acknowledgment

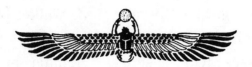

A S A DAUGHTER OF THE wombniverse, in a world that has devalued and almost obliterated matriarchy and the divine spirit of womb •man•hood, I say Ashe and Thank you to the sacred "womb•men" of all ages and times. You have been the strength and light of all women.

I would like to acknowledge my circle of sacred women who have continually given me love and support. They are a glorious tribe of beautiful spirits each with their own extraordinary gifts. To my Mentors, Sis-stars, Sister Queen, Assistants, Healers, Prayer Warrioresses, Divas, Queen Mothers, Entrepreneurs and Sages: I Thank You from the bottom of my heart for all that you have given. Claudette C. Faison, Dara E. Williams, Queen Afua, Ms. Shelly,

Barbara Jones, Qamar Herbert, Brenda Brown, Vinette Hart (kindred spirit Assistant), Dr. Edna R. Hill, Mother Hill, my Divine Daughter-Queen Nadira and of course, My Divine mother, Frezell. I give special honor and praise to my divine ancestral guide, Madame C. J. Walker on whose shoulders I stand. Ankhs and Praises to Goddesses (God-essences), female guardians, angelic beings, and ancestors who are the keepers of the Spirit of Womb•man. For all of you, I give Thanks, until eternity.

Contents

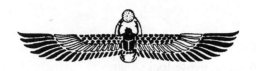

Preface

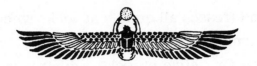

IN THIS BOOK I WILL share knowledge and information about the nature of "coiled hair"[1] and the origin of locked hair. This hair type clearly distinguishes people of African ancestry from all other people. It is my hope that the information in this book will raise the level of consciousness and empower people. My goal is to reconnect people of Black African origins to the ancient culture and spiritual heritage of their ancestors so that they may reclaim their power.

Most people know Dreadlocks as the sole context for locked hair. Dreadlocks style of hair relates specifically to a way of life that is known as Rastafarianism. Locked hair is universal. It has appeared and thrived throughout the world

---

[1] **Coiled hair** has a tight, spiral or coil formation. (Not kinky, woolly, peasy, nappy or knotty hair).

in various cultures in Africa, India, Asia, the Pacific Islands, Greece, Ethiopia (Abyssinia) and Nazareth. The texture of the hair and the customs of the people in a given region dictated the many styles and forms of hair locks.[2] Coils, spirals and tresses all qualify as locks whether they are permanently matted or loose, temporary ringlets. One style of locks, which is worn close to the scalp and in ringlets is called Pepper Corn hair. It was worn by Buddha and some of the Greeks. Another type is matted or rope hair (locks) worn by the Indian Sadhus (holy men) and the Naga Indians (Serpent People). The Shonja tribe of Africa referred to locks as string hair, because of the thin string like appearance of the hair. The Pokot tribe of Kenya wore their matted hair in a sack, much like the Rastafarians of today, and refer to them as Ancestor Hair.

Locks are universal and part of a larger cultural movement. Africa is the birthplace of locked hair and continues to be the world's oldest and greatest resource for hairlocking traditions. Across the continent of Africa, tribes such as the

---

[1] **Locks** An abbreviation for African locks.

tribes such as the Pokot, Maasai, Mau Mau, Kau, Ashanti, Fulani—to name a few—have their own unique forms of locked hair.

African people are readily identified by two features: melanated dark skin and spiraled coiled hair. Hairlocking, like many aspects of our ancient African culture, was transported across the waters with us to this country. I define and explain the hairlocking process with a focus on the origin and metaphysical meaning of locks. Once you become educated about locks, you will become empowered to make an informed choice and commitment about growing them.

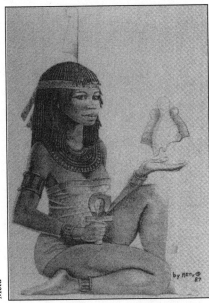

Metu

Maat Egyptian goddess who is the personification of ordered existence, harmony, justice and truth in the universe and on the earth.
See oracles of Maat on page 78.

Introduction

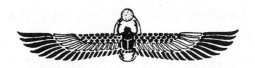

What Is Hairlocking?

Hairlocking is a biological process which occurs when naturally coiled or spiraled hair (Black people's hair type) is allowed to develop in it's natural state, without combing or the use of chemicals. The hair will go through progressive stages of interlocking and coiling similar to DNA replication, until it finally becomes a dense tight Lock; i.e., tress. The hairlocking process usually takes an average of six months to a year for completion. Once this process is complete the hair is locked and cannot be combed or loosened without being severed. -Nekhena Evans

THE NUMBER OF AFRICAN-AMERICANS locking their hair is steadily increasing. This is reflected by the growing number of hairlocking shops specializing in this service. About fifteen years ago, when African-Americans began to wear locks, people thought it was just another fad. Surprisingly, though, there has been a continuous rise in the numbers of people wearing locks. History is being made regarding natural hair care for Black hair.

In 1995 the State of New York passed legislation that dramatically altered the Cosmetology Act established over 50 years ago. The new law recognizes non-chemical treatment for hair care. Licensing is now required to perform natural hair care services. This includes twisting, wrapping, weaving, extending, locking or braiding hair. The cosmetology industry is being revolutionized by the natural hair care movement.

What has become crystal clear to me during my years of African lock grooming is that the trend towards hairlocking among Black folks is historical. We are experiencing a cultural awakening as symbolic as the trend towards the afro in the sixties.

In recent years, Africentrism has been growing, causing a cultural and spiritual transformation in our lives. People of African ancestry have gained access to information that was previously suppressed or hidden, and have begun to recognize and appreciate the significance of knowing Black history. This is reflected by the explosion of African hairstyles i.e. locks, braids and twists, the African influence on fashion and the availability of a wide selection of books written for and about Black people. In Black magazines we see more Africentric fashion, hair styles and articles advising us to return to our roots. So today, you can get the *how-to's* and *where-to's* of getting "the African look." But the question is "what is the meaning?" Given our society's preference to finding quick and easy fixes to everything, it's understandable that people of African ancestry may choose quick fixes for their hair. However, we are discovering that this might not necessarily be the best approach.

The movement towards Africentrism is not a movement towards Africentric commercialism it is due to this "awakening," an ushering in of spiritual consciousness that is revealing itself as we approach the second millennium. Many religions and schools of thought speak of the new millennium as a paradigm shift in our communication and our interaction with each other. This period will be characterized by a new and more profound consciousness developing within man and woman one necessitating that people respond from inner knowledge as opposed to external information-a shift from thinker to knower. It will be a time of planetary peace and harmony in which truthful communication and a sense of community will exist. Cultural diversity will be valued, and people will be more compassionate. As we approach the New Age, I call it the "Knew Age," people of African ancestry will have to be aware and knowledgeable. We had the Afro in the sixties, cornrows in the seventies and braids in the eighties; locks are the mantra for the nineties. Because of the highly spiritual era during the nineties, growing Locks takes on a special significance. Growing locks is a process that requires a long term commitment. Ultimately, it becomes an act of personal transformation. Throughout antiquity, in various cultures' locked hair symbolized a commitment to a separation from the world (worldliness) and spiritual development. It also symbolized Sages and spiritual people. Jesus, Buddha, Ascetics, and Initiates wore their hair locked. In some instances, it symbolized being "called" by a particular deity. Historically, in the African tradition it marked a rite of passage and exemplified one's social status within the family or group.

As we move into the "Knew Age," we are reaching back into history, to reconnect to our glorious past and move full circle into the future. I decided to write this book about our coiled hair so that people of African ancestry could understand and participate in the "Knew Age."

This book will give basic information on the nature and significance of our hair with special emphasis on locked hair. In my search I have not found much written, from a holistic perspective, on Black hair. This was rather unsettling to me because of the central role that hair plays in the lives of most Black folks. People of African ancestry come from a cultural tradition of grooming and ornamenting hair. We carried this tradition with us across the waters, and we still care a lot about our "do." Unfortunately, we have also internalized a Eurocentric perspective that teaches us that the two most significant features of our identity, our skin and our hair, are not beautiful and need to be changed.

I am committed to truth. I bequeath to you the truth about your powerful hair.

Lovingly, I am Nekhena.

MISCONCEPTION: 1

Most people who wear locks are
wearing them as a fad

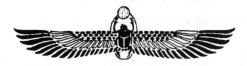

FACT

*Most people who wear locks are
committed to the hair style*

BASED ON MY EXPERIENCE OVER THE last twelve years with a wide range of clients of various ages, professions and backgrounds, I have found that most adults who decide to lock their hair have thought about it for years. Adults who grow locks are usually at a higher level of consciousness because of their personal and spiritual development. They usually have some knowledge of their African history and tradition, and are attracted to a natural living lifestyle. Generally, they have tried numerous hairstyles over the years from perms to afros and are at a point where they want to be themselves—be natural.

The decision to grow locks usually reflects an outward manifestation of a person becoming aligned with their inner being, the identity that the Creator gave them, and a readiness for a whole new way of living. Once locked, African-Americans begin a love affair with their hair.

For adolescents who choose to wear locks, there are, of course, many influences. However, the levels of self awareness and maturity varies between adolescents and adults. Therefore, the reasons for adolescents choosing to lock their 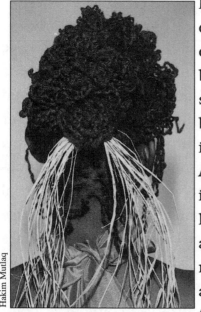 hair may be altogether different. Ultimately, it does not really matter because something is speaking to their inner being and they're wearing locks proudly. Adolescents are staying with this hair form longer than expected, and an increasing number of adolescents are wearing them since they have become in

locks are crimped and tied with rafta

Hairlocking

vogue during the last ten years.

Deciding to be true to yourself always takes courage, self-assurance and a degree of risk-taking. Making the choice to grow locks is a tremendous step because family, friends, boyfriends, girlfriends, employers, will usually try to discourage it. Some of us have bought into a way of thinking and speaking about ourselves that have kept us from appreciating our natural, god-given beauty. but this in not on a conscious level. When we wear our hair locked we become a mirror

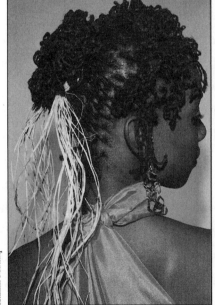

of other Black people causing them to question beliefs they have about their hair and particularly about their Blackness.

As a result of wearing locks, I have come to accept the differences and choices that we make as individuals for our chosen hair

Hakim Mutlaq

Styling and adorning is our legacy

style. Everyone must choose for themselves. It takes strength and patience to grow locks. It is a long process, one in which the individual grows emotionally, mentally, culturally and spiritually. As the hair goes through its various stages, you will find yourself becoming more attuned to these changes within yourself. Growing locks is a personal process. It is a different experience for every individual because each person has a unique hair texture. Just as a plant goes through its developmental stages, so do locks. Because of time involved, it facilitates the development of patience, self- appreciation and dignity. Your personal experiences, as well as the reactions you get from others, will also foster your individual growth.

My dream is that one day the majority of Black people (coiled hair people) will be wearing their hair in its natural state, in whatever form they choose. I hope that we continue to discover and create more designs for our natural hair because there is power in wearing our hair naturally. This power or energy is stored in the hair as a spiral. Our hair is coiled! There is an opportunity for you as a person of African-ancestry to gain an emotional, psychological, and cultural clearing about whom you are and who you can be by locking your hair. It is possible that you will experience a significant difference in yourself and in how others relate to you. You can become empowered and know your strength, just as Samson did!

MISCONCEPTION: 2

It does not matter if you refer to your
hair as dreadlocks or African locks

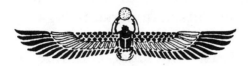

FACT

*It does matter how you name yourself; naming
creates identity*

IT MATTERS HOW YOU REFER TO YOURSELF, including
your hair. I believe people of African ancestry,
especially African-Americans, can create themselves to be what they want to be by their choice
of language. I am referring to "Nommo," the
power of the spoken word. For many of us "The
word" refers mainly to a religious context such as
the Bible. Some people relate to the importance
of "the word" in a social context, for example,
when they say, "word is bond," "word to my
mother" or "word up." Some have studied metaphysics[3] and know about becoming God-Man,
"The word made flesh." As a people however, one

---

[3] **Metaphysics-** The science that deals with matters above and
beyond the physical and material planes of existence, beyond
the visible to the invisible realms.

of our most damaging experiences has been our disconnection from our ability to relate to symbolism and the power of the spoken word

We were, and still are, deeply spiritual; deeply powerful people. In a hieroglyph we could capture the magnificence and power of a single object and the entire universe in one. We kept the spiritual gifts of understanding through symbolism-dreams, visions, the word, intuitions (in-to-it/tions). We must continue to preserve our inheritance. If we do this, even on the mundane level of keeping our word, we can claim our heritage of being a great people with many spiritual gifts.

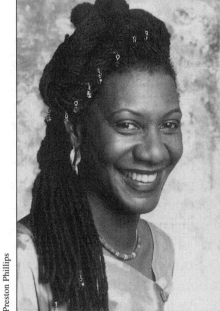

Just like "as a man/woman thinketh, so is he/she," you are your word. What you say to yourself and what you say to others about yourself is crucial. Other people's words can have a powerful effect on you. For example, when a teacher, parent or mate says something like: "you

Preston Phillips

Enlightenment of the crown with Austrian crystal adornments

are smart," "you are wonderful," "you can achieve anything." This can be empowering. It has been demonstrated, for instance that if a person is challenged in a physical contest and repeats positive statements (affirmations[4]) the results are blatantly different from when that same person repeats negative ones. In the former, the individual gains

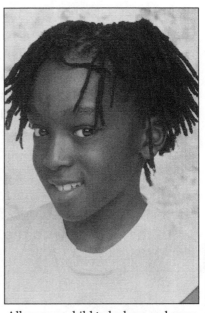

Allow your child to lock up and grow up free!

strength, while in the latter they lose strength. When you make positive affirmations about yourself and to yourself, you will attract positive results. If we can embrace this principle, the results can be miraculous.

You should know something about the origin of the word "dread." It is an Old English word that refers to fear and horror. The words "locks" or "tresses" that refer to hair, and are also of English origin. Dreadful was the term used by the English in speaking of the Africans hair when they were captured and brought to U. S. shores.

---

[4] **Affirmations-** Statements of positive truth.

I would suspect that they were referring to our naturally locked hair and perhaps sometimes to the infested, matted hair that undoubtedly developed from the horrific conditions of the middle passage. In any case, the same negative connotation that they ascribed to everything "black" was also ascribed to our hair. Black people have since come up with their own interpretations of "dread," which reflects something meaningful and positive. We have a legacy of trying to make the best out of the worst situation.

In the new millennium we must make time for a new dialogue and language. It is time that we define ourselves as who we really are: African and beautiful, brand New Bein's (Nubians[5]). We have to take more care and responsibility in what we say, and appreciate the power of the spoken word and how it helps to create our reality. Most religious or spiritual philosophies advise us on the importance of what

Preston Phillips

Silver fox/The Elder. Ancient wisdom and Beauty

[5] **Nubians-** Inclusive term denoting *All* people of African ancestry.

Hairlocking

we say and think. You know what I'm talking about, "you better watch what you pray for 'cause you just might get it," "man does not live by bread alone but by every word that proceedeth out of the mouth of God," "by thy word thou shalt be justified, and by thy word thou shalt be condemned" and "life and death are in the power of the tongue." How-to books, with such generic titles as *How to be Successful How to be a Millionaire, How to Love Yourself, How to Develop Yourself Spiritually,* all have in common a discourse on the power of affirmations (the word)-"The word links man with omnipotence." This is not mysterious, and you do not even have to memorize affirmations for them to work. If you read positive statements aloud daily from a piece of paper, you will begin to notice a difference in yourself. If you don't believe me, try it for one week and see. Tell yourself daily: "I am Perfect, I am Loving; I am Powerful." Spend time in the mirror looking at yourself and speaking these words to yourself (in the morning before you go out is a good time). See the results.

I challenge you to go back to the source, back to the African tradition for direction. Call your beautiful locked hair Nubian Locks. There is nothing dreadful about your locked hair, It is important to use language that uplifts and empowers you as well as affirms your identity and dignity.

MISCONCEPTION: 3

Locks and dreadlocks are the same.

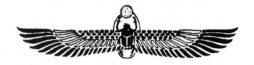

FACT:

Dreadlocks relate specifically to rastafarianism;
locks are of African origin and are global

A FRICANS HAVE BEEN WEARING LOCKS since antiquity. I encourage you to go to the library and
look at the pictures of African tribes. The Maasai
of Tanzania are a perfect example of this tradition. They are known for their extraordinary
beauty, regality, high culture and creativity. We
carry the same tradition. One of the most fasci-
nating discoveries I made was to recognize the
direct connection of Maasai hairstyles to the
extensions and locks we've seen re-emerge in
recent years.

. The gift that Rastafarians have given to
African Americans is that they maintained an
important aspect of our ancient culture, locked

hair. Without them, it may very well have been lost. We should be grateful to them. Rastafarians who know their history, appreciate seeing all their brethren wearing their hair naturally. They are clear about their African roots and embrace it.

The only distinction to be made between locks and dreadlocks is purely on a physical level. The differences are superficial at best. Dreadlocks are organic and African Locks are cultivated. What they have in common is that both are natural (chemical free), Africentric, and are usually rooted in a sense of spirituality, consciousness and cultural pride. The Rastafarians, who believe in Africentricity and naturalness (which are one and the same), believe in leaving the hair in its natural state and not doing anything to it. The Caribbean environment of hot sun, sea saltwater and fresh air (which is similar to Africa facilitated the hairlocking (dreading) process. African Americans who wear locks have the same natural affinity, but because of their unique cultural history and environment, prefer to wear it cultivated. They manicure and cultivate their locks. These come from the African tradition of ornamenting and grooming both of which have always been an important aspect of African culture. African men and women alike have historically spent a great deal of time grooming each other's hair. This was a way to be intimate and to share time and positive energy by communicating and beautifying each other.

The distinction between locks and Dreadlocks is that locks are cultivated and Dreadlocks are not, however, they are cousins and we are one people! History has shown us the strength of a united people.

MISCONCEPTION: 4

You must be Rastafarian, Jamaican or
from the islands if you wear locks

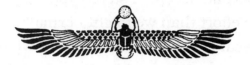

FACT:

Most people who wear locks are of
African ancestry

S OME PEOPLE ASK, WHILE OTHERS assume that
Black people, who wear locks, are Jamaican,
Rastafarian or from the islands. I mentioned ear-
lier that locks originated in Africa. One of the
main purposes of writing this book was to educate people about the facts. I am aware that the
above misconception may be based on limited
knowledge. Stereotyping does very little to
enhance communication or understanding. We
must be vigilant lest we fall prey to separatist
and limited ways of being. If you are open to
communicating and understand why a person is
wearing locks, openly ask that person why they

decided to wear Locks or what it means to them. This may be a good way to learn more about it.

We should observe how we speak to each other and how we treat each other when it comes to our hair, or anything else for that matter. Going beyond accepted stereotypes requires a little more effort than we might normally expend. It is necessary, however, that we be willing to go the extra step. We need healing. As a people, we must help and heal each other.

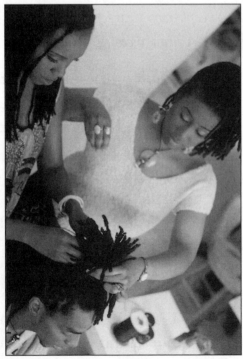

Women together in unity; styling

Hairlocking

MISCONCEPTION: 5

Hair is dead matter, a waste product
that serves no significant purpose

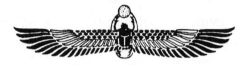

FACT:

Hair is alive and part of our Whole being

T HERE ARE THEORIES CLAIMING THAT hair is simply
dead matter. These theories view hair as a
waste product that the body throws off because
it no longer needs it. Another views hair as an
extension of the scalp that is not alive because it
has no nerves or arteries. These theories are primarily Eurocentric. This view of hair's purpose is
yet another example of the difference between a
European context and an Africentric context.
The European context tries to separate and
divide things into distinct, measurable, compart-
mentalized entities. The Africentric context sees
things as integrated, connected and holistic. It
views individuals as whole beings consisting of

physical, spiritual, mental and emotional dimensions.

It is within the Africentric context that we can say, with assurance, that hair is alive, particularly hair that is coiled. We can look at the living fibers that cover the earth such as trees and grass, as evidence that hair is alive. These elements are living, connected, interdependent parts of the ecology. These fibers are alive and organic like your hair. They require the basic cosmic food of the universe, the four elements: air, fire (sunshine) and water (moisture); you are the earth element. Your hair requires these, too. Hair also responds to atmospheric conditions of the weather and seasons. For example, winter weather usually requires that you oil your coiled hair more because it dries out. Hair also acts as a natural biofeedback system, responding to stress, thoughts, emotions and internal dietary states. Healthy hair requires a holistic approach, proper diet, positive thoughts and loving emotions.

The ancients as opposed to modern man, understood that hair has a much deeper meaning. They had more wisdom and intuition about hair. Within our crowns is housed our ancient race memory [6] and ancestral connections. Race memory refers to "the surviving intelligence of our ancestors, if a place between individual consciousness and the collective unconscious." It is sometimes called racial consciousness because, one part of the psyche may be explained through recent cause but another reaches back to the deepest layers of racial history. The conscious mind is the storehouse of human memory. The subconscious Mind is the storehouse of racial human memory and the cosmic or Divine Mind is the storehouse of cosmic memory. Our coiling hair is part of the Divine design which originated in the Divine Mind. All people are essentially made up of electric and magnetic (electromagnetic) energy. Meta-physically our hair acts as a wire conductor collecting, storing and transmitting electromagnetic energy. God gave people of African ancestry two very important gifts. These gifts allows us to absorb energies from the universe and be in greater harmony with it. They are the melanin in our skin and the coil in our hair.

---

[6] **race memory-** The surviving intelligence of our ancestors; racial consciousness imprint from past generations. Part of the subconscious mind.

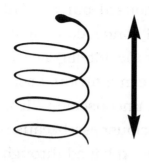

Coiled hair like a spring stores and release energy

You are blessed with a body that can enhance your ability to absorb light, information, sound, nature, or simply put—*life*. People of African ancestry have an extra facility of telecommunication ability and power because we are blessed with an airtight coiling system (antennae) at our crowns, our pinnacle. coiled hair in conjunction with melanated skin makes the entire body a vehicle of absorption and perception. It can transmit and store knowledge from outside and within. We, Black people, are in a deep spiritual realm.

So, don't let anyone fool you. Your so-called kinky, nappy, peasy, picky, knotty hair is not dead. It is alive, and it is a special blessing to you from the Creator.

Structure

Our hair is divided into two parts. The part above the surface of the skin is called the *hair shaft* and the part below the skin's surface is called the *hair root*. Both the shaft and the root consist

Diagram of hair and skin

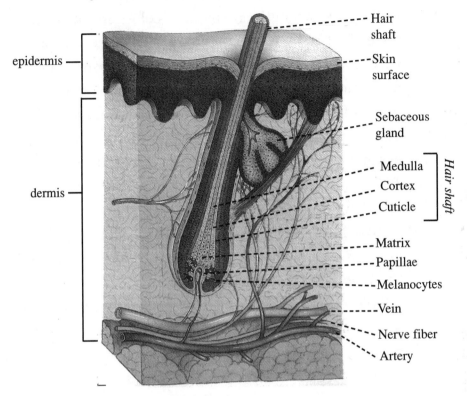

of three concentric layers of cells. The outermost layer is called the *cuticle* and consist of flat cells that are arranged like the scales on a fish and contains the hair's pigment. The layer below the cuticle is called the *cortex* and it forms the major part of the shaft consisting of long rope like cells that contain pigment granules in dark hair but mostly air spaces in white hair. This layer determines the thickness or thinness of the hair as well as its strength, resilience, color, shape and form. Soft baby like hair has a thin cortex while very coarse hair consist of thicker fibers. The innermost layer is the *medulla* and it too contains melanin pigment granules and air spaces. The medulla is sponge like and contains protein, cystine and other amino acids, water and fats. This layer also helps to determine the texture, elasticity and resilience of the hair.

The hair follicle encloses the hair root. As hair grows away from the scalp it's shape, size and thickness is determined by the shape of the hair follicle. A cross section of the hair reveals that straight hair is usually round. wavy hair is usually oval or round, curly hair is almost flat and coiled or Black hair is flat and spiraled

At the base of each follicle is an enlarged onion like structure called a bulb. The bulb has a nipple shaped indentation, the *papillae* of the hair, When you pull out a hair, The whitish end you see is part of the papilla. It contains the many blood vessels that nourish the growing hair. The bulb also contains a ring of cells called the matrix, which is a growing region of cells.

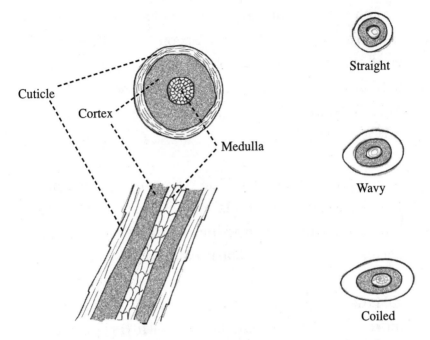

Cross-section of hair types

Cuticle

Cortex

Medulla

Straight

Wavy

Coiled

They are responsible for the growth of existing hair and they produce new hairs by cell division when older hair are shed. This replacements occurs within the same follicle.

Sebaceous or *oil* glands are generally connected to the hair follicle. The secreting portions of the glands lie in the *dermis*, which is the bottom layer of skin. The *epidermis* is the top layer that we can see and feel. These oil glands open into the necks of hair or directly onto the skin surface. Oil glands secretes an oily substance called *sebum,* which is a mixture of fats, cholesterol, proteins and inorganic salts. Sebum helps keep hair from drying out and becoming brittle, prevent excessive evaporation of water from the surface of the skin and leaves the skin soft and pliable. Sebum works its way down the hair shaft to lubricate the hair.

Color

The color of the hair is due primarily to melanin. It is synthesized by melanocytes scattered in the matrix of the bulb and passes into cells of the cortex and medulla. Dark colored hair contains mostly melanin. Blond and red hair contains variants of melanin in which there is iron and more sulfur. Gray hair occurs with the progressive decline in *tyrosinase* an enzyme necessary for the synthesis of melanin. White hair results from accumulation of air bubbles in the medullary shaft, when the production of melanin declines.

Growth

Each hair follicle goes through a growth cycle and there are three stages to this cycle. In the *catogen* stage the new hair is preparing to emerge from the hair follicle. During the growth phase or *anogen* stage new cells are added to the base of the hair root, the hair grows longer. In time, the growth of the hair stops and the resting or *telogen* stage begins. During the resting stage the matrix is inactive and the hair loses moisture and separates from the papillae. After the resting phase a new growth cycle begins and the old hair is pushed out of the hair follicle. In general the scalp hair grows for three years and rest for about 1 to 2 years. When the hair is locked it seems to defy these stages and remains in an extended period of continuous growth.

The hairlocking process also occurs in stages and there are five stages to this hairlocking (Dreading) Process:-

Stage One:

Pre-lock phase or baby locks

Stage Two:

Budding phase or teenager

Stage Three:

Shooting phase or adult locks

Stage Four:

Contracting phase or elder locks

Stage Five:

The Aging Phase.

Stage One: *Pre-Lock Phase*

This is the Lock 'Initiation' phase. The hair should be finger or palm rolled (not gel and comb twisted) into thin, tightly coiled spirals. This process is to initiate the spiraling/coiling imprint which evolves into the locking matrix. The appearance of the hair is thin, tight medusa like spirals.

This is the infancy stage we call 'baby locks.'
Phase One (baby)

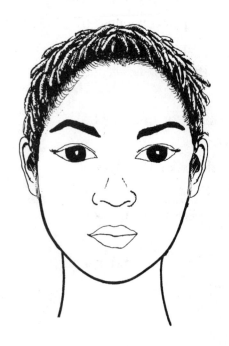

Stage Two: *Budding Phase*

During this phase the thin, tightly spiraled lock appears to explode in one spot into a bud (like a pea in a pod). The bud itself is the first indication of process. The pre-locked hair has now begun to network at the bud. This process usually occurs about three-quarters of an inch down the lock from the root. At this stage the lock is progressing and needs its space It behaves like a teenager, somewhat rebellious, has a mind of its own and need its space in discovering its own way.

Phase Two (Teen).

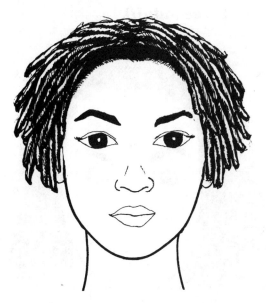

Stage Three: *Shooting Phase* (adult locks).

After the budding phase, the entire lock begins interlocking and matting, the direction is downward from the bud to the end of the hair and back up toward the scalp (similar to how some plants develop). The hair closest to the scalp is not locked; this is where you have new growth. During this phase, the hair increases its density because it begins to replicate itself like DNA. Your hair remains in this phase for the longest time anywhere from one to two years

Phase Three (adult).

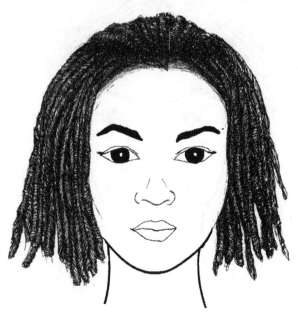

Hairlocking

Stage Four: *Contracting Phase (Elder locks)*

The hair becomes mature adult locks an airtight interlocked spiraling network system. The locks become consistent, tight and fairly solid. At this point it will probably be fairly long and the hair will grow extraordinarily, once the spiral form has been established (elder locks). Like an elder the locks are set, stable and quite uniform in their appearance.

Phase Four (elder)

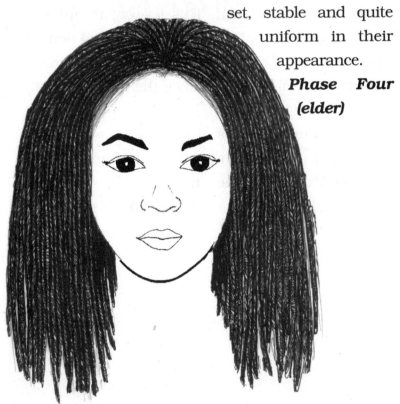

Congratulations you are now locked !

Stage Five: The Aging Phase

Finally once the locks have been established for years (about 5 years or more) The locks begin a natural process of aging just as human age physically. The aged hair looses on of its three layers overtime. This usually shows up as thinning near the ends of the hair where the oldest hair is now positioned. This level of thinning is relative to one's natural hair texture and density maintaining good hair 'healthy' management reduces thinning issues since the hair is usually pretty long at his point.

Trimming the locks at the ends is sometimes an option. Most find that with an abundance of hair at this stage they need not fret over this process. For some people thinning never becomes an issue.

MISCONCEPTION: 6

You can grow Locks fast

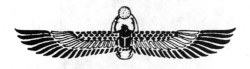

FACT:

Locks take 6-12 months to mature

GROWING LOCKS REQUIRES AN investment of time. It necessitates putting forth time, faith, patience, risk-taking, attitude changes,' going against the grain, shifting your "comfort zone" or just plain old accepting your God given inheritance. If you are looking for a quick and easy way to get "the African look" like "the Jordache look," you may be in for a surprise. Yes, people with coiled hair have the hairlocking potential or matrix within their brain computer, but it must be activated, and not with Jheri-curl activator. Your ancient race memory has to be turned on, jarred, nurtured and stirred by you. This can occur, for example, if you have your hair palm rolled into the spiral form for a time, while you

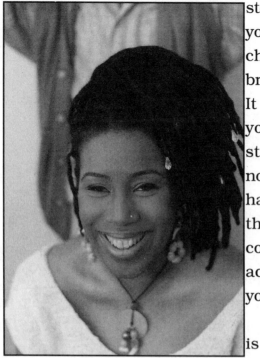

stop tearing out your hair with chemicals, a brush or comb. It can happen if you just "be still" and do nothing to your hair and allow the Creator to come in and activate it for you.

The palm roll is the most authentic and effective tech-

I am so happy I locked my hair. I love my locks

nique of starting locks because it simultaneously incorporates many essential properties. If you try what I call "the fast food method" of growing locks, which is gelling or beeswaxing your hair into locks, you probably won't get the results you desire. Although many people start their locks by either braiding or twisting (double strand twisting) their hair. These methods are not the most effective way of starting locks. They can produce the result in the end, but they skip past an important underlying process: that of the genuine spiral. A facsimile does not accomplish genuine results.

What many people fail to realize is the importance of metaphysical law. Metaphysics (meta=beyond/ physika=physical) relates to the science or workings of invisible or unseen forces. Most of what goes on in life such as in the body, mind and spirit is unseen. It is not visible to the naked eye. Although we cannot see these dynamics, they are nonetheless occurring continually. Let us look at the Pyramids for instance. The Pyramids are one of the world's greatest wonders that continues to baffle modern man. This is

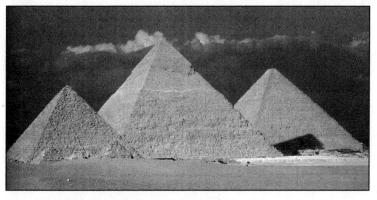

The three pyramids of Giza in Egypt Africa

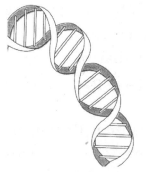

because they were built by people (Black folks) who had an understanding of the science of metaphysical laws, such as the power of numbers, shapes, forms and energy (and not just the physical laws). They comprehended that all energy and

The spiral of life itself. A molecule of DNA

power manifest according to its particular form or structure. These same laws manifest in locks. All energy is in the form of a coil, and we have the coil in our hair naturally and innately. We have the same spiral in our hair as electricity, tornadoes, whirlwinds, DNA, galaxies! These are all forms of powerful energy. It is this form that is established and reinforced in the hairlocking process. The connection to the Source is made, and hair becomes a receiver and transmitter of divine emanations.

Growing locks takes endurance and commitment. For those of you who feel you lack the strength or discipline required to endure the process I hope you will find this book encouraging. You can do it! If you can't find it within yourself to go through the process, then, perhaps, you need to further your journey in finding your spiritual self and cultural identity. Read books on the Black or African experience, personal development or spiritual growth. Attend cultural activities. Go to church. Connect with those who impress you as spiritually or culturally clear. "Seek and ye shall find." Then, and only then, will you have the inner strength to grow locks. And remember this: your hair is your crowning glory. It is the Most High part of your body. It is

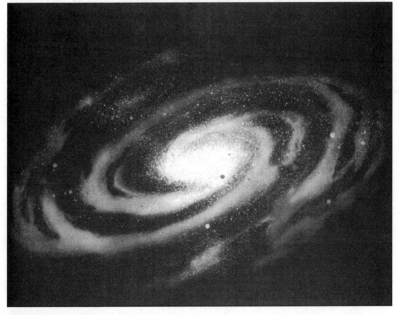

A spiral galaxy

your temple. It is your Crown Chakra Center, your power station, your computer center. This is where your life force comes in and flow out to the universe. So, be persistent and keep your head to the sky!

Locks are Nature's Power

WE HAVE THE SAME SPIRAL IN OUR HAIR AS

ELECTRICITY, TORNADOES,

WHIRLWINDS, DNA AND GALAXIES.

MISCONCEPTION: 7

All you have to do to grow Locks
is not comb your hair

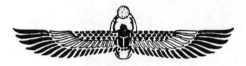

FACT:

*Growing Locks requires some work
on your part*

THIS MISCONCEPTION HAS ITS ORIGINS in the Rastafarian/Caribbean tradition but is not completely incorrect. While it is true that if you did not do anything at all to your naturally coiled hair, it would eventually lock up (it's also called matting). The phenomena of hairlocking have gone beyond this point. What has occurred with the phenomena of hairlocking, like most other life processes, is that it has changed with time developing and evolving in a positive direction which has facilitated new knowledge and choice. People can now choose to wear their locks organically or cultivated. The reasons they choose to

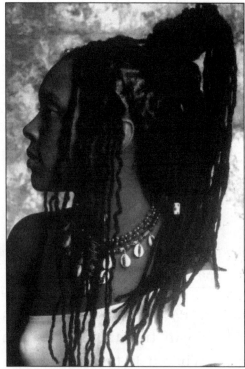
I am a Divine Queen by Divine Right!

wear them either way are based on their own values and sense of beauty. These values occur within the context of their own definitions of environmental issues such as their social, familial, work, religious spiritual, mental and physical environments.

Ultimately, the decision to leave your natural hair in either its organic state or to cultivate it is simply a matter of personal preference and choice.

MISCONCEPTION: 8

Coiled hair, Black people's hair
type, has limited growth potential

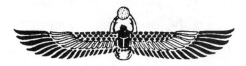

FACT:

*Locked hair challenges the accepted belief that
hair growth stops after a certain point*

THE HISTORY OF THE ANCIENTS REVEALS that the saints and sages instinctively and consciously allowed their hair to grow. One of the claims European scientists makes is that when hair reaches a certain length, it stops growing. When it comes to locks, this is not true. Black hair has limited growth potential only when it is not kept in accordance with the natural form that God gave it; the spiraling coil form. If you put your coiled hair in its correct form, your hair will not only grow but it will continue to grow. Some of you might have seen Rastafarians with Dreadlocks almost down to their feet. If you have been wondering if the Dreadlocks were real or fake, the answer is: the locked hair you saw was real; not extensions, not a weave. Continual growth will occur without exception if you lock your hair. One factor that will vary from individual to individual, however, will be the rate of growth. Generally, once the spiraling process is started, you will see a significant increase in growth rate.

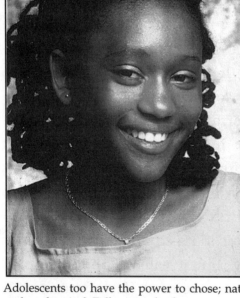

The question that comes up most when considering locking one's hair is, once I get my hair locked, and it gets long, will I be able to take it out? The answer is no. You cannot take the hair out once it is locked; you must cut them

Adolescents too have the power to chose; natural or chemical. Follower or leader

Hairlocking

off. I would suggest that the person asking this question takes a personal look at what might be motivating them to want to take out or uncoil their hair.

We must be re-taught to love our natural, beautiful selves and stop trying to be who we are not. Once we can embrace our cultural identity, we will be able to make a meaningful contribution to ourselves, our families and our communities.

MISCONCEPTION: 9

Locked hair is not versatile

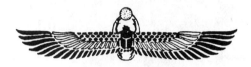

FACT:

Locked hair is quite versatile and
uniquely individual

LOCKED HAIR IS AS VERSATILE AND creative as the individual who wears it. Until recently the only form of locks worn were Dreadlocks, which are a free hanging form of locks. As more African -Americans have embraced cultivated, locked hair, the choice of styles and adornamention has expanded. Collectively, as our ancient race memory has been re-awakened by the ushering in of spirit, some of the most beautiful and creative braids, twists and locks are emerging.

Locked hair can be designed into many different styles and accentuated with natural ornaments such as gold, copper, brass, shells and crystals. These accents energize the head and

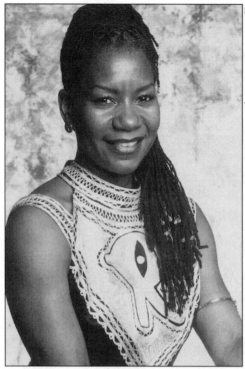
Royal Beauty! Ancient, Divine, Sublime

spirit. Locks can also be wrapped in fibers or threads in a variety of colors and textures. Like chemicalized hair, locked hair can be worn in any style. For example, braided, twisted, crimped, pinned up, rolled are all possibilities. The contrast is in the intensity, the richness and the fullness which locks present.

Locked hair has been described as "nature's first hair style" and "the ultimate in natural coiffure." If our hair is truly our crowning glory we have a responsibility to carry it. We should wear our garden of locks beautifully and magnificently however, we design it.

MISCONCEPTION: 10

Locks or dreadlocks are dirty and unsanitary
because the hair is not washed

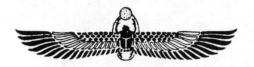

FACT:

*Virtually everyone who has Locks washes their
hair regularly*

ALTHOUGH THERE IS A DISTINCTION between
Dreadlocks and Nubian Locks, in both cases
the hair is generally washed regularly; once a
week, once every two weeks, once a month.

The natural coiled texture of most black hair,
will undoubtedly attract substances such as dirt,
lint and oil. The differences in cleanliness are the
type of maintenance, the type of products used
and the quality of the products used. One must
cultivate their hair, separate it, oil it, condition it
and remove lint from it-particularly in the begin-
ning. Using oppressive substances like beeswax,
petroleum products, heavy oils or grease,

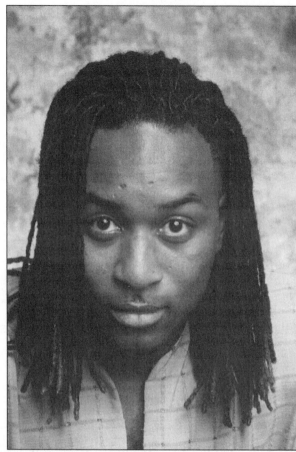

increase the probability that the lock will retain dirt and debris. Beeswax, gels, and heavy oils will give the locking effect on the exterior, however, they actually

Brothers too, are working it out

inhibit the metaphysical (unseen) and physiological processes that go on inside of the lock.

The result is it will take longer and more work to accomplish the goal of having the hair permanently lock. In addition, taking this route denies the individual. The time and experience needed to make the mental and emotional adjustments that will occur with the new physical change such as not having to do anything to fix your hair, accepting the hair's natural affinity, which is not always neat and manageable, feeling good about your new self identity; fears about being accepted, dealing with others opinions, and so on.

I suppose how one views their hair depends a lot on the frame of reference they've chosen. If you choose a European standard, as many of us try to do despite the obvious differences in our hair, you will act accordingly. For example, you may feel a strong need to jump in the shower and wash your hair daily. Given the special characteristics and needs of coiled black hair, this could prove disastrous. Additionally, frequent washings could create excessive dryness in your hair especially if restorative measures are not taken, such as conditioning and oiling. Generally, our hair absorbs a lot, just as our skin does necessitating our having to oil it more frequently. This is in contrast to straight European-type hair, upon which substances like oil and dirt sit on top of the hair. Because of its nature, it is quite appropriate for European-type hair to be washed frequently. Of course, there are exceptions. For example, some Black people have oily hair. Here, it would be appropriate for an individual to wash their hair more frequently, use less or no oil on the scalp, or use more emollient moisturizers, such as lotions, creams or conditioners.

The point is you have a choice. Part of the reason that so many of us are confused is that we have accepted European standards of beauty as the only and correct standard for ourselves. We have not been trained to name and define who we are for ourselves and by ourselves. We need to. It is time we operate from choice and freedom and not from limits and excuses.

Taking Care
of Natural Hair

IT IS EXTREMELY IMPORTANT to understand the psychology surrounding the care of an African-American natural hair. Because of the structure of Black people's hair and the substance of most European products, Black hair can be prone to dryness and brittleness. Therefore natural hair care cannot be approached with the same mindset that usually accompanies "traditional cosmetology." Many cosmetologists who use exclusively synthetic and commercial products on clients will need to alter both their approach and choice of products when dealing with natural and locked hair.

Typically, commercial setting gels, beeswax and hair glues are not accepted by the natural hair client. Clients who choose to have their hair locked expect to have simple, natural and clean smelling products used on their hair. Labels should be read carefully and the ingredients should be checked for their authenticity because many products say natural on the front label but once you read the ingredients you find it's not true. If the ingredients have too many unpronounceable items, and are combined with multiple coloring dyes like FD&C, no. 3, 4, and 5, *do not use it.* Those which list a sufficient amount of herbal and natural ingredients, with few or no synthetic ingredients, however, are highly recommended.

To properly care for natural hair, regular hot oil treatments are recommended to replenish the hair's moisture. The oil most like sebum, which is the natural oil produced by the scalp, is *jojoba.* You can find jojoba oil in most beauty supply and health food shops. You can also supplement the jojoba oil with sunflower, olive or peanut oils found in local grocery stores. Palm rolling, setting and drying the hair as individual Locks requires a natural gel product. The leaf of the aloe vera plant contains the ideal gel for setting. Aloe vera leaves can be found at most fruit and vegetable stands and must be cut and scraped for usage. Bottled aloe vera is slightly less potent, and it can be found in health food stores. Both these can be smoothed and enhanced by adding essential oils and water. The five basic oils recommended for their nutritional value to the hair are

> *rosemary,*
> *nettle,*
> *lemon verbena,*
> *lavender* and *peppermint oils.*

After the hair is dried with a hood or blow dryer, the above oils can be combined with any of your favorite

Hairlocking

scented oils for a finishing sheen.

Listed below are products that are healthy for natural and locked hair. Many of the suggested products are not made by large beauty manufacturers. With the growth of the natural hair industry, there has emerged a community of grassroots natural beauty and health entrepreneurs who are making products specifically made for Black hair. These products are usually simple, natural and have a shorter shelf life. I recommend their use because these entrepreneurs provide a high quality product. Check your local health food store for these products.

New Bein' Hair Cream/Oil and Herbal Tea Rinse, Tulani's NuCrown Hair Oil, Higher Heights Bush Butter Praise Products. Some manufactured products that work well with natural hair are:

African Formula, Cultured Oils and *Aveda*

In the '90's, natural and locked hair is challenging and transforming the prevalent standards of beauty. Black people are finally having a love affair with their hair. We can now romance our hair with the best natural living products available. Becoming a brand New Bein' means transforming beauty from the inside out.

Ten Tips

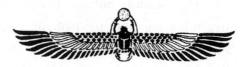

1. Do *not* use chemical or synthetic products to hold your hair together "to make it lock." i.e. gel, beeswax, lemon juice, etc.

2. Do *not* constantly twist your hair to "make it lock."

3. Once the locks are started "let them be." Stay out of them.

4. Once a week, moisturize your scalp and/or hair as indicated.

5. Do not use any product on your hair every day that includes but is no limited to oil, grease, or spray.

6. Tie your head up every night.

7. Enjoy your locks but don't focus on them too much.

8. Do *not* try to control your locks, at all times. Allow them to develop freely.

9. Get a good foundation in starting your locks by going to a professional locktician.

10. Fully enjoy the many stages of development of your locks.

Celebrate your natural hair! Love your Locks! But most importantly, *LOVE YOURSELF!*

Forty Two Oracles Of Maat
The Declaration Of Righteousness

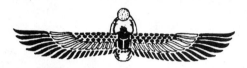

1. I *Will Not* Do Wrong.
2. 1 *Will Not* Steal.
3. 1 *Will Not* Act with Violence.
4. 1 *Will Not* Kill.
5. I *Will Not* be Unjust.
6. 1 *Will Not* cause Pain.
7. 1 *Will Not* waste food.
8. 1 *Will Not* Lie.
9. I *Will Not* Desecrate Holy Places.
10. I *Will Not* Speak Evil.
11. 1 *Will Not* Abuse My Sexuality.
12. I *Will Not* Cause the Shedding of Tears.
13. I *Will Not* Sow Seeds of Regret.
14. I *Will Not* Be an Aggressor.
15. I *Will Not* Act Guilefully.
16. I *Will Not* Lay Waste the Plowed Land.
17. I *Will Not* Bear False Witness.
18. I *Will Not* Set My Mouth in Motion (Against Any Person).
19. I *Will Not* Be Wrathful and Angry Except For a Just Cause.

20. I *Will Not* Copulate With A Man's Wife.

21. I *Will Not* Copulate With A Woman's Husband.

22. I *Will Not* Pollute Myself.

23. I *Will Not* Cause Terror.

24. I *Will Not* Pollute the Earth.

25. I *Will Not* Speak in Anger.

26. I *Will Not* Turn From Words of Right and Truth.

27. I *Will Not* Utter Curses.

28. I *Will Not* Initiate A Quarrel.

29. I *Will Not* Be Excitable or Contentious.

30. I *Will Not* Prejudge.

31. I *Will Not* Be An Eavesdropper.

32. I *Will Not* Speak Overmuch.

33. I *Will Not* Commit Treason Against My Ancestors.

34. I *Will Not* Waste Water.

35. I *Will Not* Do Evil.

36. I *Will Not* Be Arrogant.

37. I *Will Not* Blaspheme Ntr (The One Most High)

38. I *Will Not* Commit Fraud.

39. I *Will Not* Defraud Temple Offerings.

40. I *Will Not* Plunder the Dead.

41. I *Will Not* Mistreat My Children.

42. I *Will Not* Mistreat animals.

INTERTWINED
The Locked Hair Conference
Intertwined III -
"Re-Membering Who We Are"
October 1999

INTERTWINED is New York City's *First and Only* Locked Hair Conference. In Intertwined we honor the tradition of "Locked Hair" and we create a space where all people can explore their "hairitage," share their "hairstories," and respect both their inner and outer Beauty. We create a powerfully healing collective consciousness in this all day experience of inquiry, affirmation, inspiration and celebration.

intertwined is now in its third year! The first Intertwined was held on December 30, 1995. Its theme was *"A Gathering of Coiled Crowns."* The second Intertwined was held on July 21, 1997. Its theme was *"Unlocking the Future Of Locked Hair."* The third Intertwined is planned for October 1999. Its theme will be *"Re-membering Who We Are!"*

The Locked Hair Conference is multifaceted. It includes an African Marketplace, Community Forum, Panel Discussion, Documentary on "Hairlocking Traditions," a Healing Temple, Locked Hair /Fashion Show and a showcase of Entertainment.

Hairlocking

Intertwined was created and produced by Nekhena Evans, Master Locktician and the author of *Hairlocking: Everything You Need To Know*. Her business, New Bein' Enterprises specializes in Locked Hair Care and Adornment. New Bein' provides all natural Hairlocking Services and Products, Adornments for the hair and body and educational services. Intertwined is one of New Bein's educational programs which seeks to educate and empower at the community and national levels.

Hair texture and skin color are at the core of self-identity for African Americans. Historically Black hair has been portrayed negatively. This has adversely affected our sense of self and our standards of beauty. New Bein' is committed to reclaiming and reviving ancient legacies as instruments for personal and collective transformation. It is committed to continuing this tremendous healing work. This conference is about self-determination, positive self-identity, natural "be-you" ty and love.

Up to this point, there has been no fiscal sponsorship. It has been done solely through voluntary community support and love. We need your financial support to do continue this legacy into the New Millennium. Will you support this vision of Beauty?

New Where New Bein' is... "Be-You" ty is present. New Bein' transforms from the inside/out!

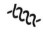

On Beauty

In the word Beauty, lies one of the most powerful realities of human existence. Indeed, it is only a two letter word yet. it is the essence of humanity and true beauty. The word is "BE," One of the most ancient paradigms of self-identity (who you are or who you be) distinguishes it in terms of three primary perspectives they are:

1) having
2) doing and
3) being.

According to this paradigm People usually value themselves according to one of these three ways of being.

1) *Have* - A person thinks that who they are is a function of what they have and the more material things they possess the more they are. Actually, they think they are what they possess. This has always proven to be false.

2) *Do* - A person defines themselves primarily, in terms of what they do. For example, they are a big executive of a large corporation, they work for a prestigious organization or business; they

have a very impressive job title, therefore they think highly of themselves based on what they have achieved.

Finally there is 3.) A person determines themselves by how they are "be-ing;" how they are being in relation to themselves, others and the world. It is here, in the domain of being that Beauty lies. It involves valuing oneself on the basis of how you are treating yourself i.e. with honor and dignity. How you are treating others i.e. family, friends, lovers. How you are treating your community. Are you contributing meaningfully to your own community? finally, how you treat the global community or planet; what is your purpose for being here and What difference will your life make to the planet? Beauty in this context emanates from "inner beauty" manifesting itself outwardly!/physically. This is True Beauty.

There are a lot of illusions that try to disguise themselves as Beauty; appearance, image, attractiveness, clothing, make-up, colored contact lenses, sensuality, popular culture, Eurocentric standards of beauty, styles, looks, etc. However, when you look Beauty straight in the eyes, Into the mirror of her soul. she will reveal that who she truly is, is who you are being In your life. Like life itself, Beauty can seem quite complex, although in essence it is very simple. Unfortunately the societal times that we live in does not support exploration or reflection into the domain of being as it once did I am continually inquiring into this whole question of Being .

Glossary

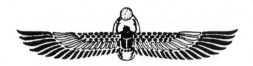

Natural Hair: Hair that is just the way the Creator gave it to you at birth. It is not altered by heat or chemicals.

Locked Hair: Hair, usually Black hair or coiled hair types, that is allowed to go through a biological process of evolution, from a spiral formation into a complex network formation, known as "locking." Once the networking/intertwining pattern is established the hair compresses, becoming an airtight, solid mass or lock.

Braid: Two sections of hair which are spiraled around each other into a twist formation, similar to rope. It is most often referred to as a two strand twist. Three sections of hair which are interlaced alternately into a flat triad pattern.

Perm: a.k.a "permanent." A misnomer describing a process of chemicalizing the hair with the alleged results of permanently straightening it. (as in never having to do it again). In actuality a permanent (application of chemicals to natural hair) does permanent and irreversible damage. It breaks down and restructures the bonds of the hair making it straight but it is quite temporary. Once you begin "perming" your hair it requires frequent "touch-ups." Perms are known experientially to have deleterious and damaging long term effects on the hair because of the chemicals.

Touch Up: Process of chemicalizing any new growth of natural hair at the roots/scalp to match the previously permed hair on the scalp. It has to be done at regular intervals (usually 2 -3 weeks) once you start "perming" your hair.

Sister Locks: A recent innovation in natural hair styling which utilizes a tool to knot the hair on itself giving a somewhat similar appearance to locks.

Dreads/Dreadlocks: A misnomer for locks, carried over from two traditions. Firstly is the Rastafarian way of life, which refers to the uncut, unmanicured locks as Dreadlocks because of the fear they instilled in the White man. Secondly, the Eurocentric tradition of England, referred to locked hair as dreadful as they have historically slandered and disempowered any cultural feature that is not theirs. Today Africans perpetuate this slander by referring to their locks as "dreads." The most accurate description of this hair form is

Locks, or African Locks which denotes its place of origin.

Spiral/Coil: The original universal form of all life as reflected in the double helix of DNA. All energy begins and resonates in this form at some level. People of African ancestry are endowed with this gift of spiral/coil on the crown of Africans to enhance their energy/spiritual interaction in life.

Hair Texture: A term describing the depth and feel of an individuals hair. Hair texture is usually described as three types: fine, normal and coarse. This distinction is based on the density and thickness of the hair. Most Black people have varying combinations of the three types in their hair.

Cuticle: The outermost layer of the hair when magnified looks like over lapping shingles on a roof.

Cortex: The middle layer of the hair determines the thinnest and thickness of the hair.

Medulla: The innermost layer of the hair.

Hair Shaft: The part of the hair that is above the surface of the skin.

Hair root: The part of the hair below the surface of the skin.

Bulb: The part of the hair that holds the matrix of growing cells and surrounds the follicle.

Papilla: nipple shape indentation at the base of the hair.

Follicle: Structure that surrounds the hair root

Epidermis: is the surface layer of the skin.

Dermis: The underlying layer of the skin below the dermis.

Oil glands: Structure that secretes sebum onto the hair and sometimes directly onto the skin.

Melanin: A brown-black pigment that gives hair and skin its color and is capable of absorbing ultra-violet (UV) light,

Melanocytes: Cells that produce melanin,

Sebum: Substance secreted by the sebaceous glands That helps to protect the hair.

References

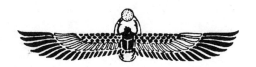

Gawain, Shakti. *Living in The Light.* California: New World Library, n.d.

Morningstar, Sayini. *Natural Locked Hair Care Booklet.* n.d.

Nessler, Charles. *The Story of Hair.* New York: Boni and Liveright, 1928.

Puryear, Herbert B. *Sex and The Spiritual Path.* New York: Bantam Books, 1986.

Scovel Shim, Florence. *The Power of The Spoken Word.* California: DeVorss and Company, 1945.

Teish, Luisah, *Jambalaya.* New York: Harper and Row, 1988.

Tepilot Ole Saitoti, with photos by Carol Beckwith. *Maasai.* New York: Harry Abrams, 1980.

The Holy Bible. Original King James Version.

Closing Statements

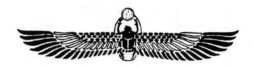

HOPE YOU HAVE FOUND this book informative and provocative. The basic premises of my philosophy are:

1. Hairlocking is an original ancient African cultural tradition.

II. Hairlocking, throughout the world, has historically symbolized spirituality, reflecting a spiritual awareness, a spiritual experience or a spiritual vow. It continues to symbolize an individual's spiritual journey.

III. Hairlocking has historic and symbolic meaning for the entire African -American community signifying a reconnection with Africentricity and spirituality.

IV. The practice of Hairlocking represents

an important cultural and spiritual tradition that requires the utmost respect in its inculcation. It must be practiced in a context of healing and holism. It is an art, and a science and practitioners known as Lockticians and Hair Naturalists must handle it responsibly.

Many practice the art of hairlocking but lack a general knowledge of the basics. There is a need to address the historical, cultural and spiritual aspects of Nubian Locks, because many people do not have this information and want it. It would be a benefit to both clients and practitioners to have the basic knowledge, values, standards and ethics, so that everyone involved has the same understanding. Values set the foundation for the commitment and the quality of services to be provided. Standards set a consistent level of expectation of services and treatment. Ethics provide a balance for the framework to guide the practice.

It is my hope that one day all lockticians:

1. Are qualified and trained to become practitioners and educators in all aspects of hairlocking including its origin, its history, its meaning, and its practice.

2. Utilize a holistic and Africentric perspective for working with clients thereby preparing to work on many levels-physical (practical), mental, emotional, spiritual and cultural.

3. Provide services in an environment that is physically, emotionally and culturally nurturing to clients.

4. Provide services in a highly respectable and professional manner.

5. Provide clients with information on maintenance.

6. Are available for follow up consultation, and support clients concerns regarding their locks.

7. Use products that are natural and healthy.

These are just a few possible suggestions to start with.

Lastly, I leave you with this simple yet profound truth stated by the ancient African philosopher Imhotep. It has inspired me to write this book and continues to urge me on:

To Thine Own Self Be True!!
Peace and Love. .

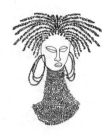

New Bein' Enterprises

invites you to try
Our All Natural Hair Care System

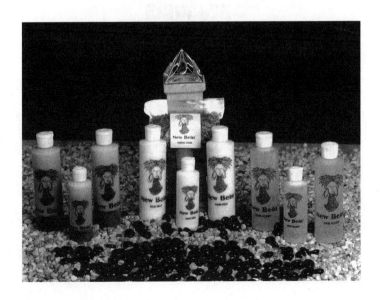

Everything You Need To Know

**New Bein'
starts
maintains
styles, and
colors locks**

**New Bein' offers consultations
natural hair jewelry natural hair care
products
body temple adornments**

**New Bein'
provides 100 % natural service.
New Bein' transforms from the
inside out
call (718) 636-5725**

94 ❖ *Hairlocking*

New Bein' Enterprises
Pioneers in Natural and Locked Hair Care!

THE NEW BEIN' ALL NATURAL HAIR CARE SYSTEM

Black hair is distinguished by its unique coiled shape. This unique form has very special needs. The most important need of coiled hair textures is moisture. New Bein' has created a line of all natural hair care products designed to meet the unique moisture needs of naturally coiled hair textures. *The New Bein' All Natural Hair Care System* is a complete regimen for healthy hair of all types.

New Bein' Herbal Moisturizing Shampoo

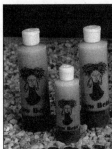 New Bein' Herbal Moisturizing Shampoo is a *final shampoo*; it is used on the final wash. Our shampoo is so effective that it does not matter what kind of shampoo you use for your initial washes. New Bein' shampoo is infused with loads of herbs and moisturizers, which restore the moisture that is stripped by commercial shampoos.

Directions:

After you have washed your hair with the commercial shampoo, use a small portion of New Bein' Herbal Moisturizing Shampoo for the final wash. You don't need much as it is so rich! Condition your hair as usual. You will notice the immediate difference in how your hair feels.

New Bein Hair Milk (Inner Moisturizer)

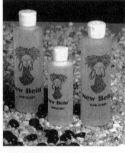

New Bein' Hair Milk is a perfect match for the moisture needs of coiled hair textures. It replaces grease, which tends to be too heavy, attracting lint and dirt. It provides deep inner moisture while maintaining a light natural finish. New Bein' Hair Milk soothes the scalp, creating balance and calming itching. New Bein' Hair milk is excellent for removing braids (extensions) and for making any texture of natural hair manageable. It can also be used for starting locks. New Bein' Hair Milk is a Kiss to your scalp and hair!

Directions:

Apply New Bein' Hair Milk directly to the scalp and hair about once a week (or as needed). It is so rich and creamy you can go lightly with it!

New Bein' Hair Honey (Outer Moisturizer)

New Bein' Hair Honey is the complement to New Bein' Hair Milk. It is a feather light blend of natural and essential oils based in shea nut oil. New Bein' Hair Honey provides outer moisture or sheen. It is not like most heavy oils, which tend to clog the pores and create build up.

Directions:

Use New Bein' Hair Honey when the hair appears dry or dull. For the best results, use New Bein' Hair Honey in conjunction with New Bein' Hair Milk alternating between the Hair Milk once a week and the Hair Honey about 34 days afterwards. It will lift the hair, giving it a light, beautiful sheen.

Hairlocking

HERBAL TEA RINSE AND CONDITIONER

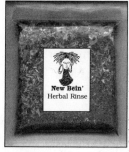

New Bein' Herbal Tea Rinse and Conditioner is a blend of over 25 herbs that are specifically for healthy hair and scalp therapy. It can be used as a toner to strengthen the overall hair health or to eliminate scalp problems such as dandruff and itching. One package of New Bein' Herbal Rinse and Conditioner makes about three usages.

Directions:

As a Conditioner.

Bring two cups of water to a boil. Remove from heat. Add one heaping teaspoon of New Bein' Herbal Rinse and cover. Allow the tea to steep for about 10 minutes and then strain. Pour the tea through the scalp and hair and leave in. For extra strength catch the tea and pour it twice.

As a Toner.

Follow the above directions and then pour the tea into a spray bottle. Spritz onto the hair as needed. New Bein' Herbal Tea Rinse and Conditioner will condition and strengthen the hair constantly.

New Bein' Enterprises
• P.O. Box 400106 •
Brooklyn • NY • 11240-0106 •
• (718) 638-5725

NEW BEIN' TRAINING SERVICES

Nekhena Evans is the author of the nationally acclaimed book, *Hairlocking: Everything You Need To Know*. She is a Master Locktician, in the practice of Hairlocking for over ten years. Nekhena is the proprietress of New Bein' Enterprises, a business committed to 100% all natural Hairlocking services, education, empowerment, transformation and "Be-You"ty for the mind, body, and spirit. Nekhena Evans is now offering training classes in:

The Art. Science and Tradition of Hairlocking

Hairlocking Training will be offered in three modules:

1) **Intensive I (One Day Training)** - A one day group training specifically designed for those who are experienced in the hair care profession.
2) *Intensive ii (Two Day Training)* - A two day group training designed for those new to the hair care profession.
3) *One-On-One Training* - An intensive individual training designed to meet your specific individual needs. Training consists of Theory and Hands-On Practice. Schedule to be arranged conveniently. Begins when you are ready.

Intensive I

(One Day Training)

This training is designed for those who are experienced in the Hair Care profession. The focus is primarily on the Hairlocking Business and training in Hairlocking skills. The cost for the Intensive One Day Training is $500.00.

The training is from 10 a.m. to 7 p.m. Trainings are usually held on Sundays.

Intensive II
(Two Day Training)

This training is designed for those who have no experience with professional hair care in any setting. Intensive II is a comprehensive two-day training in all aspects of Hairlocking, from the Hairlocking business to practice. Day one will consist of a comprehensive wholistic introductory course on Hairlocking.

Day two will consist of Hairlocking Skills and Practice. The cost for the Intensive ii Two Day Training is $600.00. Trainings will usually be held on the weekend (Saturday and Sunday) or on two consecutive Sundays.

ONE-ON-ONE
(Individual Training)

This training is designed for anyone interested in receiving Hairlocking training independently (without a group). It will be tailored to meet the specific needs of the individual. An agreement of time/schedule will be arranged between the teacher and student. The cost for individual training is $500.00.

There is a $100 non-refundable registration fee for all trainings. All balances of payment are due two weeks prior to the training date. No personal checks are accepted, only money orders or cash.

All training materials are included in the training fee. Additional New Bein' products will be available for purchase on the training date.

To receive an application call (718) 638-5725. State your interest.in one of the three types of training described as possible with the $100 registration fee to secure your place as classes and space will be limited.

Everything You Need To Know

NEW BEIN' VIDEOTAPES
Lock Styling & Lock "Mane"tenance

INTERTWINED- New York City's First Locked Hair Conference
The Locked Hair Show - $19.99
Features 6 Lock Shops.
Taped at Long Island University on December 27, 1995.

LOCKED HAIR MANE-TENANCE - $19.99
Nekhena Evans presenting.
Answers most common manetenance questions.
Taped at Lucille Roberts in Brooklyn, N.Y. June 1, 1997.

LOCKED HAIR STYLING AND FASHION SHOW - $19.99
Features 5 lockticians demonstrating styling.
Taped at the Victoria VI Theatre in Harlem New York, September 27, 1997.

TAPE	COST	QUAN	TOTAL
Locked Hair Conference	19.99		
Lock-Mane-tenance	19.99		
Lock Styling/Fashion	19.99		
Sub Total			
NY Resident add			
8.25% Sales Tax			
S&H (See shipping chart)			
Total Cost			

Hairlocking

You're invited to visit our Website at:
www.new bein.com
You will be able to see all of our Products
including the Hair Adornments online.
You can send us e-mail
at:
Locktician @ aol.com
Tell A Friend !
E-MAIL THEM OUR SITE ADDRESS.

COMING IN OCTOBER 1999
INTERTWINED New York City's THIRD ANNUAL
LOCKED HAIR CONFERENCE
"RE-MEMBERING WHO WE ARE"

It is is an event you don't want to miss!
Stay tuned for details!

Call us to pre-register. Send in $20.00 to reserve
your place. The conference will take place in
Brooklyn,
Tentative date Oct. 16,1999

Everything You Need To Know

NEW BEIN'

INNOVATORS OF NATURAL AND LOCKED HAIR

New Bein' is the creator of many firsts in the Natural and Locked Hair Care Industry!

In September 1993, New Bein' wrote the first book on Hairlocking *Everything You Need To Know Hairlocking.*

In May 1994, New Bein' introduced their own line of all natural *Natural Hair Care Products. New Bein' Hair Milk, New Bein' Hair Honey* and *New Bein' Moisturizing Shampoo.* These products are designed specially for coiled hair textures.

In July 1994, New Bein' created "HAIR-RINGS" a new concept in hair adornment for those who wear their hair in locks, twists and braids. Hair Rings are beautifully handcrafted beaded hair jewelry in special designs or with ornamentation. They are unique in that they adjust to fit all sizes of hair.

In May 1995, New Bein' introduced two new lines of Natural Hair Jewelry, *The Cowrie Queendom* and *Crystal Light Jewelry.* These are beautiful hand-crafted cowrie shells, plain cowrie shells with Austrian crystals, and Austrian Crystal hair jewels with a special press on and off feature for easy wear.

In December 1995, New Bein' sponsored New York City's First Locked Hair conference, "INTERTWINED -A Gathering of Coiled Crowns. "

In June 1997, New Bein' sponsored the Second Bi-Annual Locked Hair Conference "INTERTWINED-Unlocking The Future of Locked Hair." The next conference is being planned for October 1999.

Currently, in 1998 New Bein's latest creation is *Body Temple Adornments' sacred jewelry inspired by the ancient legacy of Kham*, the first civilization. These beaded necklaces, bracelets and earrings, feature ancient Khamitic symbols. Special to the Body Temple Adornments, is The *"Menyet" Collection—necklaces reserved for the goddesses"* according to the Khamitic legacy. These are inspired designs that are truly one of a kind pieces.

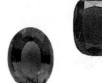

CRYSTAL LIGHT JEWELS
Natural Hair Jewelry
for Locks, Braids and Twists

Crystal Light Jewels are made of the finest imported crystal-Swarvorski. Swarvorski Crystals are renown for their crisp, clear, brilliant shimmering colors, and bright sparkle. *Crystal Light Jewels* are designed for easy wear in your natural hair because they are easy to attach and can be worn for any length of time. Simply press the two-prong hook into the lock, braid or twist. Gently pull the prongs apart to remove it. Adding just one Crystal Light Jewel to your hair adds drama, energy and beauty to your crown!

OVAL	CUBE	DROP	TEAR	SLEEK	FLAT DISC	SIZES
						Large Small

Sizes: Large and Small
Cost: $ 5.00 per small crystal and $ 7.00 per large crystal

Colors	Shape	Size	Color	Shape	Size
Clear	C, P, R	(S,L)	Golds		
	FD, O, S	(L)	Aurum	P (one size	M)
Blues			(solid color)		
Capri Blue	R	(S,L)	14 kt Gold	P	(S,L)
	O	(L)	(inside)		
Sapphire	R	(S, L)	light Topaz	R	(S, L)
Montana Blue	FD	(S, L)	Topaz	R, P	(S)
Reds:				FD	(L)
Garnet	R	(S, L)	Pinks:		
Siam	R	(S, L)	Rose	R	(S, L)
	P	(L)	Light Rose	R	(S, L)
Greens			Purples:		
Emerald	FD, R	(S, L)	Amethyst	R, P	(S, L)
Peridot	P	(S)	Light		
Chrisolite	P	(S)	Amethyst	R	(S, L)
Yellows:			Ambers		
Jonquil	P, R	(S, L)	Mint	R	(S, L)
			Colorado		
			Topaz	R, P	(S, L)
			Champagne	P	(S)

Hairlocking

New Bein' Enterprises
Natural Hair Jewelry
Order Form

Qty	No.	Description	Unit	Total

Name:_____   subTotal: _____

Street: _____   Sales Tax: _____

City_____St: _____ Zp _____   S&H _____

Card Type: _____   *(See below)* _____

Card Number: _____   Total _____

Signature _____   _____

Merchandise Subtotal   Shipping & Handling charges

$ 25.00 and under..........................$ 3.95

$ 25.01 to $ 50.00......................$ 5.95

$ 50.01 to $ 75.00......................$ 7.95

$ 75.01 to $ 100.00....................$ 9.50

$ 100.01 and over ....$ 10.95

MAIL CHECK OR MONEY ORDER TO:

New Bein' Enterprises
P.O. Box 400106
Brooklyn, New York 11240-0106 (718) 638-5725

New Bein' Enterprises
Natural Hair Products
Order Form

Product.	Size	Cost	Quan	Total
Hair Milk	2 oz.	$ 5.00		
Hair Milk	4 oz.	$ 10.00		
Hair Milk	8 oz.	$ 15.00		
Hair Honey	2 oz.	$ 5.00		
Hair Honey	4 oz.	$ 10.00		
Hair Honey	8 oz.	$ 15.00		
Shampoo	2 oz.	$ 4.00		
Shampoo	4 oz.	$ 6.00		
Shampoo	8 oz.	$ 10.00		
Sweat -shirt	L - XL	$ 20.00		
T-Shirt	L - XL	$ 20.00		
Canvas Bag		$ 15.00		
Herbal Tea Rinse	2 oz.	$ 9.00		
Hairlocking Book	2 oz.	$ 9.95		

Name:_____   subTotal: _____

Street: _____   Sales Tax: _____

City_____St: _____ Zp _____   S&H _____

Card Type: _____   *See below* _____

Card Number: _____   Total _____

Signature _____   _____

Merchandise Subtotal   Shipping & Handling charges
$ 25.00 and under...........................$ 3.95
$ 25.01 to $ 50.00.......................$ 5.95
$ 50.01 to $ 75.00.......................$ 7.95
$ 75.01 to $ 100.00.......................$ 9.50
$ 100.01 and over ....$ 10.95

MAIL CHECK OR MONEY ORDER TO:
New Bein' Enterprises
P.O. Box 400106
Brooklyn, New York 11240-0106 (718) 638-5725

New Bein' receives many requests for Lockticians nationally. In order to meet the demand for high quality, professional hairlocking services we are establishing the:

New Bein' Network

Let us connect you directly with clientele in your area.
New Bein' Network members receive special benefits:

Consulting Services

Training Opportunities

Products

Publicity

And most importantly

REFERRALS!

Call

(718) 638-5725

to receive information about the network

Growth & Prosperity!

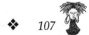

Nekhena Evans will now share her gifts with you by offering her services to you in the following ways:

Day of Adornment/Pampering Day

Offer your clients a day of pampering, beauty and adornment by bringing together healers and service providers. Possible services to be included would be pedicures, manicures, facials and massages. Ms. Evans would be able to do a presentation on "Locked Hair Care and Adornment." "Natural 'Be-You'ty," or an agreed upon topic in the domain of Beauty, Natural Hair, Self-Identity. Africentricity or related topic. The charge for the services and other details can be worked out between parties based on factors such as space, number of participants, number of service providers, etc.

Consultation Day

Ms. Evans will make herself available for a day in your space to render Locked Hair Consultations. As many pre-arranged appointments as possible would have to be made in advance (30-minute consultations of $20.00 each). Marketing planning can be discussed.

Book Signing

Ms. Evans would be available to do a book signing in any of the local, community, independent or Black-owned bookstores. This would entail either a one - two hour engagement-presentation.

Arrangements to be worked out between parties.

Slide Presentation/Documentary

Ms. Evans has produced a remarkable historical slide presentation, which documents various indigenous tribes throughout the world who instituted the Hairlocking tradition. The focus of the presentation is on the historical, spiritual and cultural origins of Hairlocking. This kind of presentation is probably most suitable for a cultural or historical organization i.e. cultural center, museum, or community based organization.

Maintenance

Ms. Evans would conduct a two-hour session on *How To Cultivate and Maintain Locks*. All New Bein' products would be made available for purchase, which would include the hair care products as well as the natural hair jewelry.

One Day Training

Ms. Evans can do a full day of training in your salon/space on *Hairlocking Theory & Practice*. The training would be (4-6 hours) (10-4pm). It would have a minimum of 7 trainees and a maximum to be determined. The cost for the training would be $250.00 per person, which is a 50% discount rate. For out of town events considerations of room and board, transportation and support staff assistance, would have to be made.. Also promotional marketing would also need to be included in the plans. All services can be tailored to meet your salon or organizations specific interest and needs. To discuss further call:

(718) 638-5725

Index

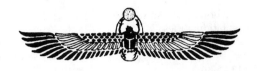

Everything You Need To Know

Notes

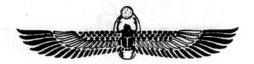

Notes

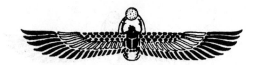

Hairlocking

Notes

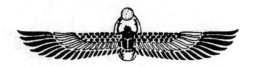

Notes

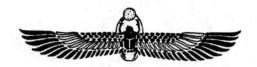

Notes

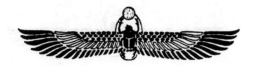

Notes

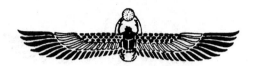

Hairlocking

Notes

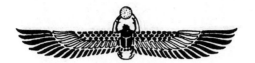

Notes

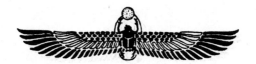

  Hairlocking